Herbal Medicine Explained

I0417486

A Guide to the Healing Power of Natural Herbs

RON KNESS

Contents

Disclaimer

We hope you enjoy reading our report however we do suggest you read our disclaimer. All the material written in this report is provided for informational purposes only and is general in nature.

Every person is a unique individual and what has worked for some or even many may not work for you. Any information perceived as advice by must be considered in light of your own particular set of circumstances.

The author or person sharing this information does not assume any responsibility for the accuracy or outcome of your use of the content.

Every attempt has been made to provide well researched and up to date content at the time of writing. Now all the legalities have been taken care of, please enjoy the content.

See your healthcare professional before starting any diet, health or exercise program!

Introduction

Herbal medicine has existed for many centuries. For much of history, it was the only medicine; in some cultures, today, it still is.

The Internet has certainly helped the ever-increasing resurgence of interest in herbal remedies for treating a huge range of conditions and diseases.

Only a couple of decades ago, patients were reliant almost solely on their general practitioner for medical knowledge. While some were prepared to consider "alternative therapies", many were very conditioned to their own education, which was strongly rooted in surgery and pharmacy as the main treatment options.

Now, patients and sufferers can do their own research, and more reassuringly, read the experiences of others with similar problems. This has allowed them to learn what has worked for others. It has also opened their eyes to the problems that some pharmaceutical "solutions" have caused individuals.

Western medicine research has made some great advances in improving human health, but it seems too obvious sometimes that certain elements have conspired to prioritize financial returns over healthful outcomes. Big pharmacy is a big industry with a lot of clout.

For some people and some conditions there may be no other viable option. For most however, it is in the very best interest of their long-term health to explore natural, herbal solutions to their conditions first.

Herbs for health is not a punchy slogan, it is a truism.

Origins of Herbal Medicine

Since the dawn of time, herbs and specific foods have been utilized by civilizations all over the world for their medicinal properties. Early cultures relied on both ingesting and topically applying plants for their healing properties.

Ancient Egypt

The slave workers of ancient Egypt were given portions of garlic on a daily basis in order to help them fight off any infections and fevers that were abundant during those times.

The ancient Egyptians are reputed as being the first civilization to write and make records about herbs and their beneficial properties. There are records dating back to 1500 BC, kept by the priests, who utilized herbal medicines including cinnamon and caraway.

Roman and Greek Origins

As ancient Romans and Greeks invaded other countries, their doctors absorbed knowledge regarding local medicines used in that area. Through their travels, their doctors also introduced the benefits of herbs such as Rosemary and Lavender to other cultures.

Chinese Medicine

Traditional Chinese Medicine also known as TCM, has been around for thousands of years. In this system, the TCM practitioner holds the wrist of their patient in a specific way and feels their pulses. They also inspect the patient's tongue, eyes and skin and then prescribe specific herbs.

Many people who have not had success with Western Medicine procedures have found great relief with this method. Aspects such as Acupuncture, Herbs, and Qi Gong exercises may be employed as part of the TCM protocol. However, herbs remain as the main medicine prescribed.

Celtic Medicine

It is believed that in Scotland and Wales, Celtic Healers and the Druids relied on an oral tradition of herbal medicine knowledge, mixing religion and rituals into the healing process.

British Medicine

In Britain, herbal medicine became abundant with the establishment of numerous monasteries around the country. Herb gardens were grown at each monastery to be used by the monks as well as the local populace.

Native Medicine

Prior to European settlers, local native cultures relied on the plants and animals in their region for their survival. Regardless of the region, the majority of cultures all over the world sourced specific local plants that aided in healing wounds, adding nutrition, and soothing the skin, muscles and bowels.

Of extreme value were antiseptic and cleansing herbs and those which provided a relaxing effect to the system.

Herbal Medicine Today

Herbal medicine works with the entire body system to help solve the root cause of the illness. This is why many remedies may need to be taken for up to 3 months before some people notice a difference.

Of course, depending on the ailment, many people may begin to feel the beneficial effects right away.

There is no miraculous wonder pill with herbs; herein lies the beauty and for some, the frustration. Instead, the whole lifestyle of the patient is taken into consideration prior to an herbal remedy treatment.

This means that during a consultation, not only the presenting symptoms such as headache and fatigue will be discussed.

Diet, sleep patterns, stress factors and bowel habits will all be taken into consideration in order to help paint a complete picture of the patient's problems.

This will allow correct selection of the necessary herbs to enable the body to regain balance and stimulate healing.

Herbal medicine seeks to be holistic, therefore the goal is to treat the cause and not only the symptoms.

The belief is that temporarily curing the body of an ache or pain or illness, but not removing or getting to the root cause, will very likely allow the issue to occur again in the future.

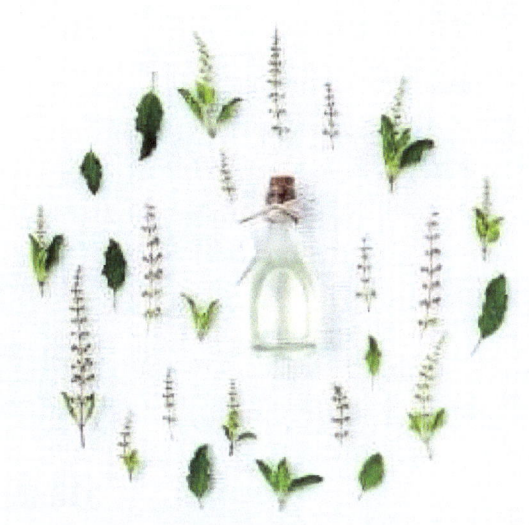

Herbal Use Explained

What exactly does 'herbal' mean? It has become a catch phrase employed by everyone from pharmaceutical companies to cosmetic companies. Many people prefer natural health and healing benefits as opposed to relying on chemically prepared products, so they look for products marked as 'herbal'.

Herbal typically refers to any kind of preparation that is derived from a medicinal plant. This broad definition encompasses any preparation made from roots, leaves, bark and flowers.

How Do People Use Herbs?

Internally

There are numerous ways to employ the benefits of herbal treatments. They may be taken internally in the form of a pill, tincture, or liquid extract. These can be purchased pre-formulated, or you can purchase the ingredients and do-it-yourself.

You can use a mortar and pestle and purchase empty gelatin capsules and grind up your own preparations to make your own pills. Be sure to research the dosage and only use organic herbs from a reputable source or those you have grown yourself.

Herbal teas can be a wonderful addition to your health as well as your daily pleasure. There are herbs which will help you feel invigorated and awake while others can help you achieve a relaxed and mellow state.

There are also herbal oils that are taken internally. Some of these are suitable for flavoring homemade toothpaste and mouthwash or taken diluted as a gargle.

Externally

When taken internally, liquid extracts, teas and tinctures are absorbed faster than pills since they do not have to be first broken down by digestion.

However, many herbal practitioners believe that any kind of liquid is absorbed more efficiently when applied externally.

Applying the herbs directly on the skin topically bypasses our stomach acid and gets the nutrients where they are required quicker. Of course, not all herbal preparations are available in a liquid format, so ask questions when you shop and look closely at the shelves to see the different options available for the extract of your choice.

External applications generally provide soothing relief while they are delivering the medicinal benefits to be absorbed via your skin. Topically, herbs can be applied as a salve, cream, lotion, oil, or poultice. You can usually even use some tincture directly on the skin if that is all that you have.

Foot baths, sitz baths or full body baths are another way to enable your skin to drink up the goodness offered by these amazingly beneficial plants. These can also be great methods for treating hemorrhoids and increasing the circulation in the body.

An herbal facial steam inhalation can be extremely beneficial for alleviating symptoms of asthma, bronchial problems and the common head and chest cold.

Adding some tea bags or oats to your bathwater can stop itching and calm rashes. Chamomile tea bags cooled and placed on the eyes will reduce the redness and inflammation of conjunctivitis. There are a host of ways to use herbs in a topical manner.

Aromatherapy essential oils are a different class of incorporation again. These are applied externally, but inhalation can provide the fastest path for achieving either relaxing or stimulating effects. These wonderful oils can provide benefits not only to physical health but to state of mind and to appreciation of pleasure.

Benefits of Herbal Medicines

There are very real benefits to using herbal medicines. First, they are all natural and have little or no side effects which makes them a healthy alternative to mainstream medicines. There are also more specific benefits that can make herbal medicines far superior to over the counter or prescription drugs.

Here are a few reasons why they can benefit you and what you can do to get the most advantage from them.

Natural Healing

Herbal medicines work by invoking the body's natural healing abilities. The natural compounds found in herbal medicines tap into the body's biological healing systems to enable and promote self-healing.

Some of the active compounds found in herbal medicines stimulate different hormones in the body. This hormonal activation helps the body to heal both emotionally and physically. These hormones, once activated and working efficiently, send specific messages to the parts of the body that require healing. The emotional aspects of disease and ill-health are often not adequately addressed by mainstream medication options.

Improved Immunity

Herbal medications are well known for their ability to support and strengthen the immune system, which is constantly being compromised by dietary and environmental inputs. Herbs contain natural antioxidants and nutrients that are helpful for improving the body's overall state of health.

By fortifying the body's innate defense system, the use of herbal medicines leads to a stronger immune system. This puts the body in a state capable of fighting against many different types of disease-causing pathogens.

Relief from Chronic Conditions

Herbal medicines can be used as long-term treatments for chronic conditions without the concern of suffering from unwanted side effects. This reassurance in itself is a huge benefit of using herbal medicines.

It has been shown that many herbal remedies work more effectively than conventional drugs in treating chronic conditions.

Back pain is one example. Taking traditional pain killer medications can cause terrible side effects, plus there is a very real risk of addiction to many drugs, including readily-obtained over-the-counter painkillers. The acute pain may be temporarily eased; however, the cycle of pain continues. This is why it is termed chronic pain.

Herbal medicines address the 'pain center' and heal the actual cause. In many cases of chronic back pain, inflammation is the root problem. One herbal remedy that can attack the root cause – the inflammation – is Bromelain. It is non-addictive, has bonus health benefits and it works for many sufferers.

Combining herbal medication, the avoidance of sugary foods and the elimination of junk and processed foods will go a long way towards providing lasting relief from chronic pain caused by inflammation.

Fewer Side-Effects

It would be wrong to say that herbal medicines do not have any side effects, however they have far fewer than mainstream medicines, and they are not as long-lasting. Some herbal remedies may have side effects and therefore these herbs should not be used without the strict supervision of a professional. If used correctly many potential side effects can be avoided, unlike conventional drugs, which even when prescribed by a licensed physician can incur unavoidable consequences.

Other Benefits

Other advantages over mainstream drugs are:

- Herbal medicines can mostly be purchased without the need for a prescription.

- You can grow many of your own medicinal herbs.

- If you are suffering from a medical condition and you either don't want to try any conventional treatments, or they are too expensive, you may have the choice of using natural medicines.

There are many more benefits than listed here, depending on the illness or disease at hand. Therefore, you may want to explore your natural options first before submitting yourself to more invasive or expensive forms of treatment.

Lifestyle Changes

Herbal medicines work much better in conjunction with an improved lifestyle. Natural remedies are not a substitute for bad lifestyle choices, but then no medication really is.

For example, herbal teas are often used as an herbal medicine. One example is Chamomile tea. It helps soothe and relax and assists people with anxiety. However, if the anxiety sufferer continues to drink excessive amounts of soft drinks and caffeine, the benefits of drinking chamomile will be limited, compared to someone who acts positively to reduce the intake of stimulants.

This is partly why you may occasionally hear a person say herbal medicines don't work. They don't experience the benefits because they don't change their lifestyle habits to support their healing.

Herbal remedies work with healthy dietary habits to bring about long lasting health benefits. This will greatly help to reduce the risk of many of the lifestyle diseases that too many take for granted today.

Herbs for Anger

Every day we are faced with challenges or situations that can make us feel angry. Some people don't have a problem dealing with these challenges while others easily become angered and emotionally out of control.

Anger management techniques vary widely in both application and effectiveness. What works for one person may not work as well for another.

Some people choose medication; however, this is often little more than something to dull the senses. As well as basically reducing sensory inputs (and subsequently quashing feelings of "being alive") most products have other unwanted side-effects.

For those people, specific herbs have healing properties that may prove to be more beneficial in helping them to manage their feelings of anger, without the side effects. Here are a few of those herbs.

Vervain

Chinese traditional medical practitioners use this herb for treating the symptoms of depression, however, it can also help with anger.

The doctors highly recommend that this herb be used with honey, and that it is used consistently. You cannot just drink one cup of vervain tea when you feel like it. For this herb to be truly effective it must be taken consistently, such as at least 2 or three cups of tea each day.

This should be done for a couple of weeks to stimulate the process of detoxifying the body of accumulated toxins, which play a part in triggering negative emotions such as anger. Chinese practitioners believe that a strong emotion, such as anger, is held in the gallbladder. Therefore, by detoxifying the body with the help of the vervain herb, anger will eventually subside and be less likely to recur.

Dandelion

Dandelion is an herb that many people turn to when needing support for problems in the liver. You may consume dandelion either as a tea or tincture.

When feelings of hostility, resentment, bitterness and anger are building up, your liver is affected and dandelion can assist to restore balance. It contains active compounds that cool down the liver, helping to regulate symptoms of anxiety, anger and other damaging emotions.

Many who use dandelion claim that its active properties work in clearing out their negative patterns of behavior. These patterns of behavior will almost certainly be contributing to the development 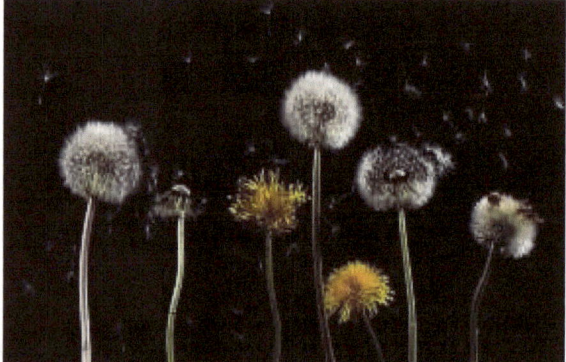 of negative emotions that includes anger.

Marshmallow Root

If you are too upset and angry to eat, take some marshmallow root. Marshmallow root positively impacts your nerves and digestion, and helps prevent feelings of anger and depression.

If you haven't had it before, you'll love its nutty flavor. It also works to help your body absorb water, which is great if you are dehydrated. Dehydration will certainly add to crankiness, anger and other negative symptoms.

Rosemary

Rosemary is known for its ability to boost circulation in the body. Chinese practitioners believe that with improved circulation an individual will find an increase in love and other positive emotions. A healthy circulatory system has a huge impact on the heart and keeps it strong against negative emotions, such as anger and depression.

If your anger is caused by adrenal burnout, it is even better to use rosemary in combination with another herb called borage. These two herbs will work together to help heal your adrenal glands.

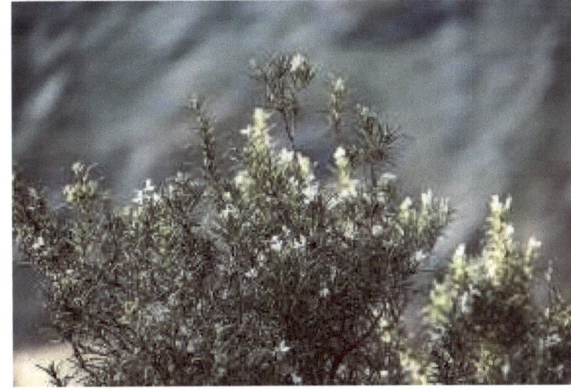

It can be very difficult not to feel irritated and angry when your health is compromised. Improving physical and emotional health with natural herbs can help buffer against negative emotions.

Herbs for Anxiety

Many of the distressing symptoms of anxiety can be naturally eased with the use of herbs. Herbal remedies for anxiety work similarly to some medications prescribed today. It is possibly more correct to say that some synthetic medicines try to replicate the behavior of herbal medicines that have worked well for centuries.

If you are looking for a natural solution to dealing with anxiety symptoms, you may find these herbs provide relieve with less side effects.

Passionflower

A team of experts conducted a study which compared the effectiveness of passionflower and a benzodiazepine drug in relieving the symptoms of anxiety.

The results showed that Oxazepam, a benzodiazepine drug used for anxiety, was found to be quicker at providing relief, however towards the end of the study passionflower and Oxazepam were found to be 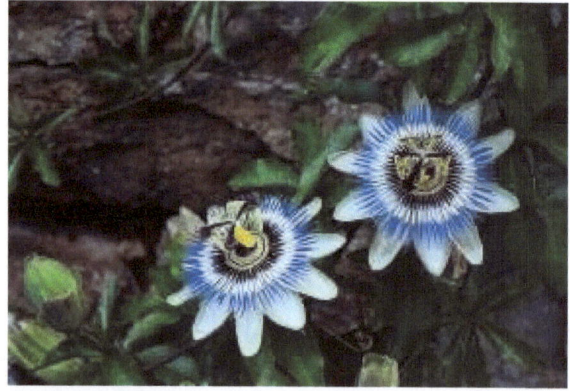 equally effective at addressing the symptoms of anxiety.

Passionflower was a little slower initially but just as effective as a remedy over the course of the treatment. Additionally, passionflower was a clear winner when it came to side effects, as it doesn't have any, unlike benzo drugs.

A separate study showed that patients who took passionflower before undergoing surgery were less anxious than patients who did not take passionflower.

Passionflower extract has shown no adverse effects on either muscle activity or mental processes.

Lavender

Lavender is prescribed by many natural health professionals for treating anxiety. Research on lavender reveals that lavender works just as effectively as Lorazepam for providing relief from anxiety.

It also shows no potential for being addictive and is useful for many other health problems arising from an anxiety disorder, such as insomnia, migraine, nervousness and restlessness.

Valerian

Valerian is commonly prescribed as a sedative. It is a popular herbal supplement for providing relief from anxiety symptoms. Valerian can help reduce physical and mental tension.

Valerian root contains valerenic acid which enhances the effects of GABA or gamma-aminobutyric acid, a naturally occurring hormone. GABA can help promote feelings of relaxation which reduces and alleviates stress and anxiety levels.

These are the same effects that are experienced after taking prescription benzodiazepine drugs.

St. John's Wort

Most people with an anxiety disorder would have heard about the benefits of St. John's Wort. The active elements of this herb are found to work effectively in treating the symptoms of depression. Anxiety and depression often go hand-in-hand and the two disorders have overlapping symptoms. Taking St. John's Wort can be helpful in providing symptom relief for both conditions.

St. John's Wort has active compounds that are helpful in prolonging the action of serotonin in order to improve an individual's mood. This is why this herb is used as an anti-depressant and for overcoming low moods.

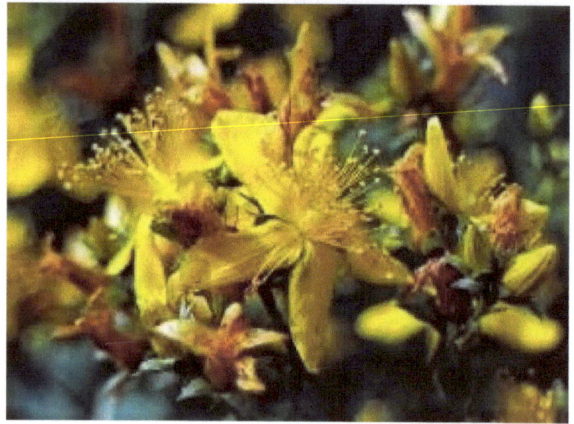

Chamomile

Chamomile is another herb used for anxiety relief. It is used to treat anxiety, stress and depression. Chamomile is known as the relaxation herb. It soothes and relaxes the troubled mind.

The effectiveness of chamomile in treating the symptoms of anxiety was studied by experts from the University of Pennsylvania. They found study participants taking chamomile for eight weeks reduced their symptoms of anxiety whereas those participants in the placebo group experienced no reduction in their symptoms.

Another study published in the *Journal of Clinical Psychopharmacology* also showed that chamomile extract therapy can be helpful for mild to moderate generalized anxiety disorder or GAD.

Lemon Balm

Lemon balm can be helpful for alleviating the symptoms of anxiety and stress. It is most commonly used for relaxation and easing sleep problems.

Herbal medicine experts say that lemon balm is more effective when used with other herbal agents. There are many anxiety supplements available which contain combinations of herbs that work well together to increase their effectiveness for providing anxiety relief.

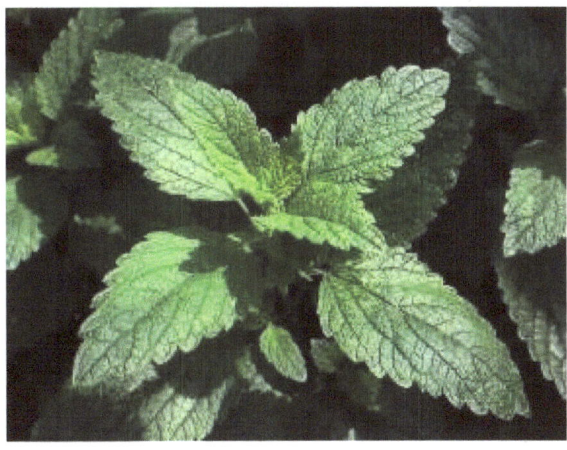

Herbs for Arthritis and Joint Pain

Losing weight is one of the best remedies for arthritic and joint pain, as it takes undue pressure of the joints. Additionally, a healthy and effective weight-loss diet will mean less intake of toxins that cause or add to the problem.

However, this can be easier said than done for some people, which is why other remedies or solutions are sought after.

Although over-the-counter pain relievers may be helpful in the short-term, long-term use can harm the kidneys and other organs. As much as possible, it is safer to opt for the natural route. This includes using herbs for fighting against pain and inflammation.

Here are a few herbs to try:

Nettles

This herb contains iron, phosphorous, magnesium, calcium, protein and beta carotene. It also contains vitamins D, A, C and B complex. Many arthritis sufferers claim that fresh nettle greatly reduces their pain and inflammation.

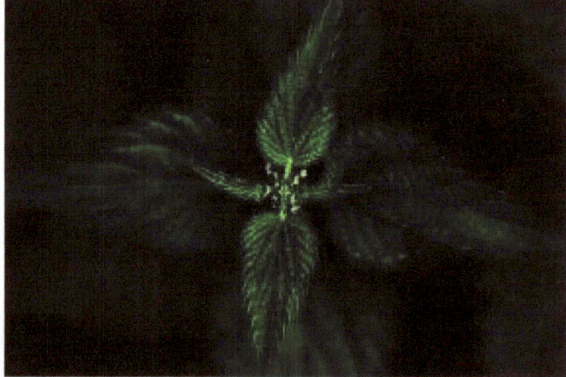

If you are currently taking NSAIDs for your arthritic pain, you might consider adding nettle to your treatment plan so you can lessen the reliance on these pharmaceutical anti-inflammatories.

Willow Bark

Long before aspirin was discovered, there was willow bark. Willow bark contains salicin, an active ingredient with effects similar to that of aspirin.

A study published in the 2013 issue of Phytotherapy Research reveals that willow bark contains active properties that can reduce inflammation. When experts administered willow bark extract to almost 500 study participants, who were suffering from rheumatic pain, the patients reported significant reduction in their symptoms.

Although willow bark is available in capsule form, many suggest that its tea works better for just about any arthritis pain.

Burdock Root

One of the best things you can do for yourself if suffering from arthritic pain is to increase your consumption of essential fatty acids. In addition to oily fish and other foods that contain these fatty acids, burdock root can also be a good source.

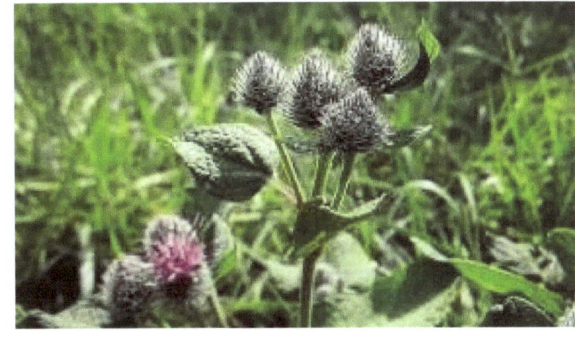

Burdock has long been a trusted herb when it comes to treating painful joints. Burdock can be taken as a tea, or used in tincture or extract form. Burdock is also being used as an ingredient in many homeopathic remedies today.

Turmeric

Turmeric is an anti-inflammatory powerhouse and has become a favorite for treating joint pain. Its ability to provide relief from arthritis pain is attributed to its curcumin and curcuminoids which are natural chemicals that can reduce inflammation.

Many arthritis patients claim that turmeric works as effectively as the anti-inflammatory drugs prescribed for them. It is used in many natural herbal supplements for helping to eliminate pain.

Experts recommend that for greater pain relief, turmeric is best taken in tea form. Turmeric capsules are also available and of course the powder can be added to cooking.

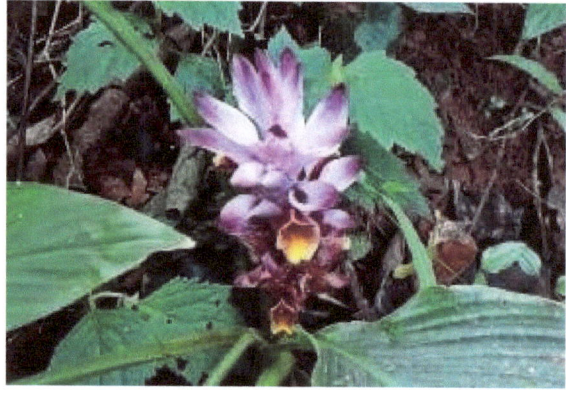

Juniper Berry

Juniper Berry has been used for treating many joint-related illnesses. The diuretic properties of this herb make it a perfect remedy for arthritis and gout, in which fluid retention causes much of the pain and discomfort to sufferers.

Juniper can be easily applied as an ointment or taken as a tea. However, some practitioners say that this herb should not be taken orally for more than a month at a time, otherwise the person can risk having kidney problems.

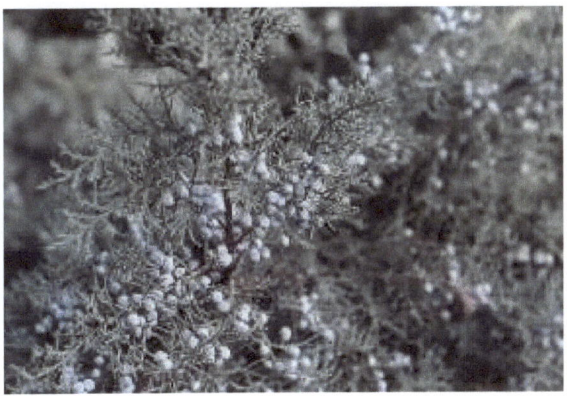

Boswellia

The boswellia herb is also referred to as frankincense or Indian frankincense. This herb has gained a good reputation among alternative medicine practitioners for its ability to fight and protect the joints against inflammation. It is believed to also inhibit leukotrienes, which attack the healthy joints of people who are diagnosed with autoimmune diseases.

There are many proven herbal remedies available to try for relieving arthritic and joint pain. Many treatments will include a combination of some of the herbs listed above.

Herbs for Headaches

If you experience headaches, don't forget to look at the psychological aspects of your pain. Some headaches stem from psychogenic issues such as depression, anxiety or stress.

If you are experiencing a vascular headache, it will more likely be eliminated with the use of over the counter analgesics. A headache caused by psychogenic issues can be more difficult to find relief from the pain. This can cause excessive intake of painkillers; whose effect is little more than "mind-numbing" if this is the case.

If the type of headache you have has emotional causes attached, rather than trying to get rid of it with over-the-counter products - that probably won't help much – you will probably find better relief from using herbs.

Whether your headache is caused from emotional stress or physical stress, it is always better to opt for natural remedies first, as taking medications only masks the pain, rather than treating the underlying cause.

The following herbs will prove to be helpful for people who are prone to headache pain, including migraine headaches.

Willow

The ability of willow bark in providing relief for headaches started back as early as the 1800s. Its active ingredient is salicin. Today, there is a synthetic version of salicin, known as salicylic acid. This product we all know, is aspirin.

This synthetic version of salicin has been found to be irritating to the lining of the stomach, which is why many people still turn to the original willow herb for treating their headaches.

It has been proven to be extremely effective against pain and fever, which is why they found a synthetic version in the first place! So this herb provides the pain-reducing effect of aspirin, without the negative side effects.

Butterbur

This herb is commonly used for treating the symptoms of migraine. Its effectiveness in relieving migraine headaches has been documented in headache journals.

One of butterburs great benefits, besides being good for treating current headaches, is that it also works to prevent the recurrence of future migraine attacks. Studies have also shown butterbur to be effective in treating cluster headaches.

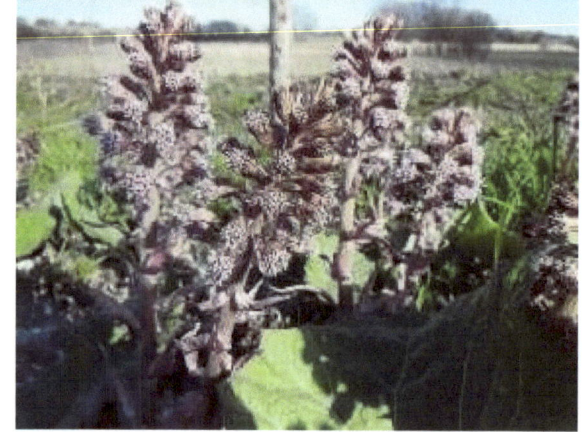

One clinical trial conducted by the Albert Einstein College of Medicine had 245 migraine sufferers as their study participants. The results showed that 68% of these participants experienced a 50% reduction in their symptoms after using butterbur.

Feverfew

Its active compounds called *parthenolide* have been found to provide anti-inflammatory effects, which also prevents the production of chemicals that cause spasms in the blood vessels.

A study headed showed that feverfew helps reduce pain and light sensitivity while also alleviating nausea. For these reasons, many people also use it as a preventative medicine for migraine attacks.

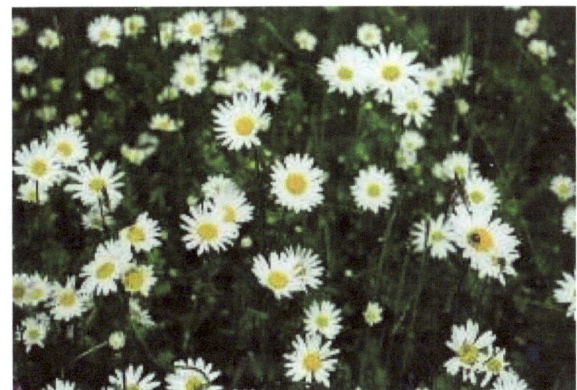

Passionflower

Passionflower is famous for its calming and pain-killing properties. By soothing the nervous system, it calms emotion and helps lower anxiety levels which can trigger headache pain. The ability of passionflower to relax the mind keeps symptoms of headaches at bay.

Drinking a cup of passionflower tea before bedtime will ease headache pain and bring on a more restful state, to allow better quality sleep.

Herbs for High Blood Pressure

High blood pressure is not a disease but rather a sign that there are problems with your health. This is why BP measurement is one of the primary diagnostic tools used by general practice doctors.

If you have high blood pressure levels, you can be at risk of developing serious heart diseases, if left unmanaged and/or untreated. The two biggest contributors to high blood pressure are poor diet and stress. When these are combined, the results can be very damaging and sadly, even lethal.

You can quite often very effectively reduce your high blood pressure naturally, by changing your diet and lifestyle habits.

As part of a dietary solution, there are herbs that can assist your fight against the effects of high blood pressure and also better keep it within healthy levels.

Hibiscus

Many people from different cultures all over the world have been using hibiscus to naturally lower their blood pressure.

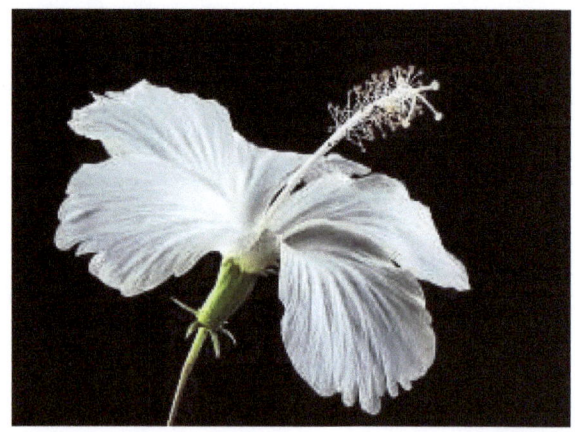

However, it is only a decade ago that experts conducted a study regarding the effectiveness of hibiscus. The results revealed that hibiscus acts effectively as a diuretic. This helps remove excess sodium from the body, which results in reduced pressure in the arterial walls.

Another finding from studies about hibiscus is that it is capable of mimicking ACE inhibitors. The ACE or 'angiotensin converting enzyme' inhibitors is a substance commonly found in pharmaceutical drugs manufactured for lowering blood pressure, and helps the body maintain fluid balance.

Basil

This herb not only goes well in many dishes, it also helps to reduce high blood pressure and has antiviral and antibacterial properties.

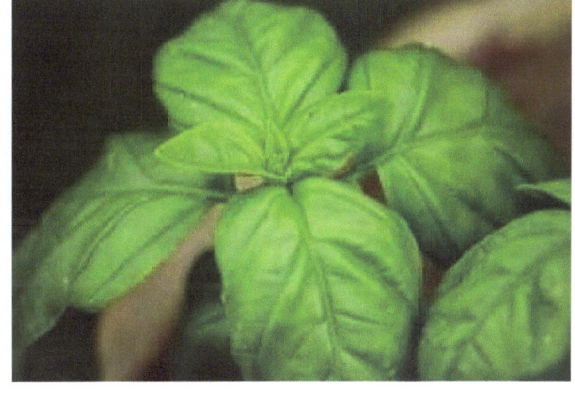

It has also been found effective for lowering blood sugar levels, while easing tension and acting as a general detoxifier.

This herb that has many health benefits and is worth adding to your list of must have herbs!

Ginger

Ginger has been used as a medicinal herb for centuries. It heals and promotes good health throughout the body.

It is excellent for improving blood circulation, which is important for healthy blood vessels and assisting in lowering high blood pressure.

It is easy to add ginger to many foods or eat on its own, so this herbal remedy is an easy inclusion in your diet.

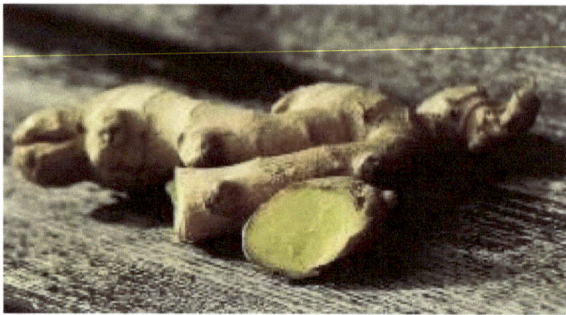

Cat's Claw

Although its name sounds like something a witch would put in a cauldron, this herb is helpful in lowering high blood pressure. Its ability to lower blood pressure is attributed to its active compounds which work to dilate the blood vessels, thereby allowing a better blood flow.

It also functions as a diuretic which is helpful for lowering the levels of sodium in the blood, and has healing properties that support the body's natural defenses against many other diseases.

Indian snakeroot

This herb has been used for thousands of years to treat heart health problems.

Its ability to lower blood pressure is due to its high content of alkaloid reserpine which is beneficial for improving heart functioning.

It also relieves symptoms of anxiety, stress and depression which are conditions that can also trigger and sustain a rise in blood pressure.

If you need to do something about your blood pressure levels, why not start with a natural dose of herbal goodness? As discussed, these herbs have physical and emotional actions on the body's wellbeing. You'll no doubt find that other areas of your health improve at the same time if you do!

Herbs for Insomnia

Are you on occasion having a hard time getting a good night's sleep? Or worse, would you class yourself as suffering with chronic insomnia?

If so, a few good herbal remedies might be just what the doctor ordered, or possibly should have. Here are a few for you to trial until you find what works for you. Sleep is critically important for good health and longevity, so don't ignore bad sleep patterns.

Valerian

Valerian is commonly used as an herbal sleep aid and calming agent.

Patients who use valerian root have claimed that they have experienced a shortened length of time to fall asleep, their sleep duration has 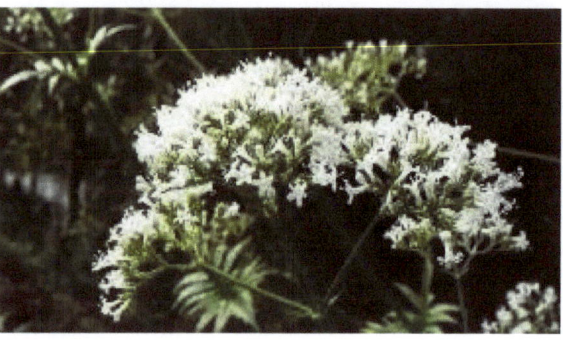 increased and their sleep quality improved.

Valerian capsules are available and normally taken at least one hour before retiring. Reports reveal that its effects last for approximately four hours.

If your poor sleep patterns have become habitual, you may find yourself waking during the night. Instead of lying awake for hours, you can take another dose of valerian.

This will help develop new sleep patterns, by keeping you relaxed and asleep.

Chamomile

Chamomile is perhaps one of the most famous herbal sleep aids. Many studies have proven the ability of chamomile to help people who have chronic insomnia as it acts as a mild sedative.

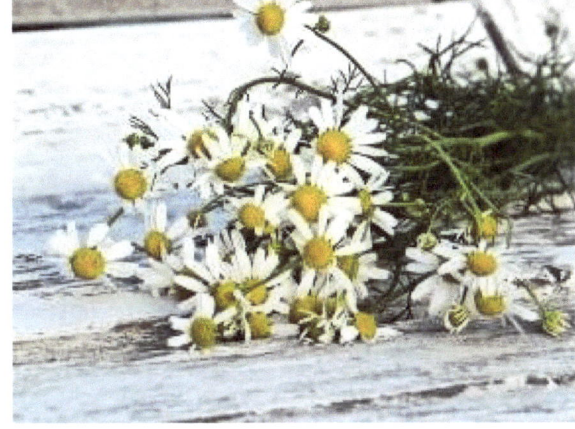

The studies have shown that chamomile helps promote sleep by allowing the person to first experience mental calmness, which also helps reduce the symptoms of generalized anxiety disorder.

Most chamomile users drink a cup of chamomile tea before bed if they need to get a good night's sleep, or ease their anxiety and built-up tension. The properties in chamomile help with deep relaxation.

Lemon Balm

The power of lemon balm to effectively help people fall asleep has been recognized for centuries. Lemon balm has been a favorite go-to herb whenever insomnia strikes since the Middle Ages.

Its clean, refreshing smell brings on a relaxed feeling. You can add a few drops of lemon balm to your pillow to help ensure a restful night's sleep.

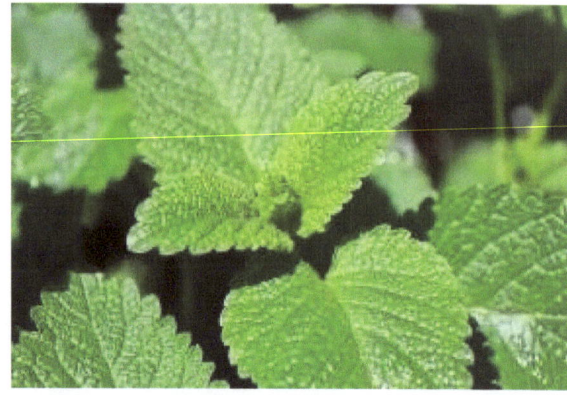

If you are a little skeptical, and think that a few drops of lemon scent won't work, give it a try before you doubt its sleep-inducing abilities. A study published in the **Neuropsychopharmacology Journal** showed that lemon balm may indirectly influence sleep and relaxation by first making some improvements to a person's mood.

In addition, lemon balm is also referred to as nootropic herb because of its brain-enhancing effects, and is known to improve cognitive performance.

Schisandra

Although not as common as chamomile or valerian, schisandra is another herb which has earned a high reputation among Chinese medical practitioners, due to its remarkable ability to induce relaxation.

The schisandra berry is capable of producing potent sedative effects and helps increase sleep duration.

Experts agree that this herb shows great potential in helping people who are suffering from insomnia, and more study on this herbal remedy will be forthcoming.

Schisandra is considered an excellent herb to use for improving all-round health, due to its vitamin and mineral content, and has been called a "superfood".

One or All?

Now you've read about a few herbal remedies you can use for insomnia. You can start by making a calming cup of tea, or go all out and take a few valerian supplements and add a few drops of lemon balm to your pillow before bed too.

Let's see if one or all of those things helps you get a good night's sleep! How much difference would that make to your day?

Herbs for Lowering Cholesterol

If you have been diagnosed with high cholesterol levels, it's quite probable that your doctor advised that you begin taking statin medications. However, you may be a person who is opposed to taking these types of prescription medications for various reasons. If you are one of these people, you will be happy to know there are natural herbs that can help lower cholesterol levels naturally.

Skullcap

A study conducted by Japanese researchers showed that skullcap can help the body reduce LDL (bad) cholesterol and also boost the production of HDL (good) cholesterol.

Skullcap benefits the body in many other ways too. For example, it works as a pain reliever because of its analgesic properties. Skullcap helps balance your body's hormones, while stimulating the release of endorphins (your feel-good hormones).

People who are suffering from nervous disorders can also benefit from taking skullcap, due to its soothing effect on the nervous system, making it useful in preventing seizures and other spasmodic reactions.

Indian Gooseberry

Indian gooseberry is highly praised by traditional Chinese medical practitioners for its natural 'hypolipidemic' agent that reduces lipid concentration build-up.

Gugulipid

This herb is native to India and is derived from the resin of the 'mukul' tree. Gugulipid is known for its cholesterol lowering properties, and has been used for many years. Its effectiveness in preventing the accumulation of bad LDL cholesterol in the blood has already earned it a high reputation. Many people claim it works just as effectively as statin drugs, but without any negative side effects.

Curcumin

This herb is a member of the ginger family, and just like any other types of ginger, is known for its antioxidant properties. Curcumin is helpful in fighting high cholesterol levels as it prevents the absorption of cholesterol in the intestines. The conversion of cholesterol into bile acids is increased and the excretion of bile acids is stimulated by this potent and powerful herb.

Garlic

The potency of garlic in boosting cardiovascular health has been proven time and time again. Cardiologists recommend the use of garlic in improving heart health. Garlic is not only a powerful antioxidant, it is 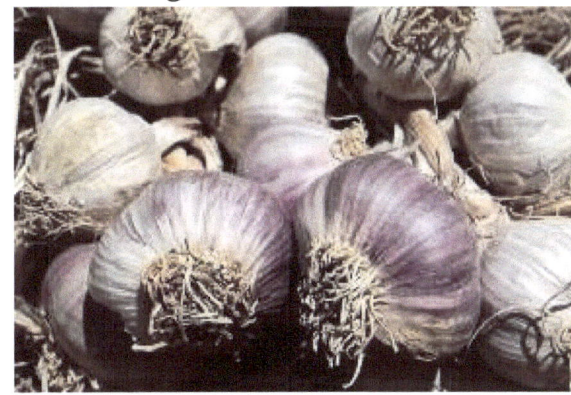 also a very effective blood thinner.

Many medical practitioners promote garlic for its ability to reduce the production of triglycerides, and garlic is also known to work as effectively as mainstream pharmaceutical drugs in lowering blood pressure.

Hawthorn

This herb is used for treating a variety of heart health problems. Hawthorn helps people who are having issues with an irregular heartbeat, chest pain, high or low blood pressure and increased cholesterol levels.

Its active compounds have been shown to help break down fats. Researchers claim that hawthorn plays a key role in lowering low density lipoproteins (LDL cholesterol) and triglycerides.

Therefore, the regular intake of hawthorn can significantly help lower a person's risk of developing cardiovascular disease.

Natural is Safer

Many of these herbs are found in cholesterol lowering supplements, so if natural treatments are for you, it won't be too hard to change to a treatment that suits you. Natural herbal supplements are safer than statin medications and don't give nasty side effects.

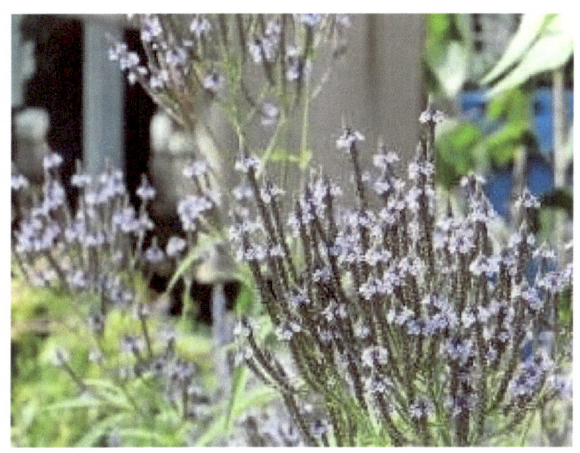

Herbs for Skin Healing

The skin is the largest organ of our body. It consists of multiple layers that protect the body against bacteria and other disease-causing environmental toxins. Adhering to a nutritious diet is one of the keys to having healthy skin, on and in all layers.

Unfortunately, some people's immune system is compromised, thereby making their skin susceptible to infection and disease.

If you experience skin problems, don't turn to over-the-counter preparations right away, give your skin a chance with natural solutions. Nature has a lot to offer when it comes to protecting and accelerating the healing process of your skin.

There are many herbs that have proven to be helpful, such as the following:

Lavender

Lavender contains linalool that aids in the healing process of several skin conditions. The same compound is responsible for the prevention of tissue degeneration and this helps reduce the signs of premature skin aging.

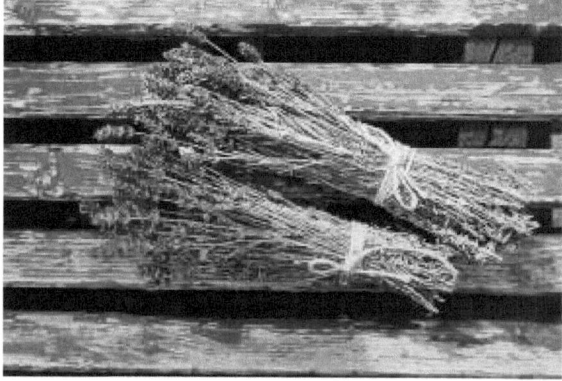

Lavender also assists in the growth and development of new skin cells. This is made possible with the help of its cytophylactic properties.

If your skin is looking coarse, dry and inflamed due to environmental toxins, lavender will certainly help as a skin salve. Lavender is known to have powerful antioxidants that protect the skin against the adverse effects of these types of toxins and pollutants.

If you are constantly stressed, this can result in rough skin, and the calming properties of lavender will both serve as your skin's shield and provide you with a sense of calm.

Calendula

The blossoms of calendula are beneficial for skin healing while also acting as a mild astringent. Research shows that calendula has antiviral, antifungal and antibacterial properties. One very appreciated quality of calendula is its ability to heal even the most sensitive skin gently.

Many people use calendula in treating diaper rash, chapped lips, minor bruises, minor cuts and burns.

Others use calendula as a facial wash to help them get rid of their acne.

Gotu kola

Researchers investigating the qualities of gotu kola found that it can treat some skin problems due to the herbs natural compounds, referred to as triterpenoid saponins. These active compounds in gotu kola were found to be responsible for not just strengthening the skin, but also for improving blood flow to the skin.

Aloe Vera

Aloe Vera is a very well-known remedy for applying to many skin conditions. If used in its purest form, aloe vera helps speed up the process of healing.

Aloe vera can be used for treating minor skin infections, burns, wounds and cysts. There are studies which indicate that aloe vera can also be used for other more serious conditions such as psoriasis, canker sores, genital herpes, dandruff, skin ulcers and eczema.

Echinacea

Although Echinacea is more popular for boosting the immune system, it is also an excellent herb for treating skin problems. Native Americans use Echinacea for healing skin 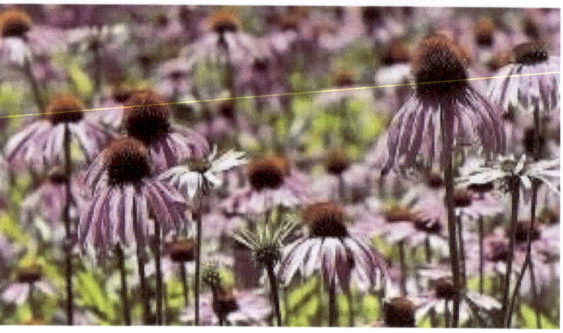 wounds, snake bites and insect stings.

There are scientific studies which have also proved that Echinacea extract possesses anti-inflammatory properties. Echinacea contains collagen protective properties that protect the skin against free radical damage.

Other studies suggest that Echinacea contains enzymes that are capable of keeping the 'skin jello' intact by inhibiting the spread of toxins, while also preventing fluids leaking from the skin tissues.

In addition, Echinacea has antifungal and anti-bacterial properties, so this herb provides benefits on many levels.

If you have any type of skin problem, check to see if there is an herb or herbal treatment to overcome it. You may even have one growing in your own garden.

Herbs for Weight Loss

Weight gain is compounded by numerous factors, however in almost all cases the major contributor is the excessive intake of food, especially of certain food types.

Eating the right foods will be the key to your weight loss success so you must be diet-conscious when choosing them. There are even herbs which can assist weight loss. These herbs act in different ways so review the following to see how you can best benefit from including them in your weight loss program.

Cinnamon

Cinnamon serves as an excellent inclusion to your weight

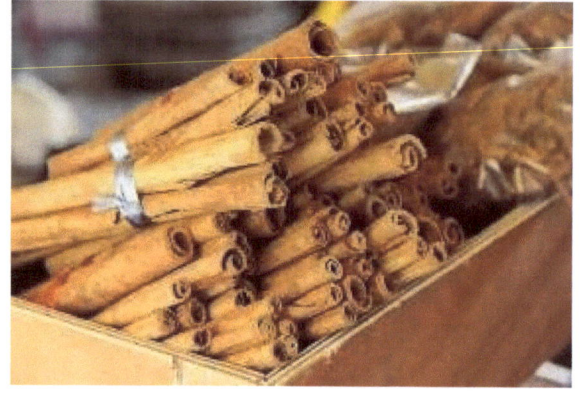

loss regimen for it helps you lose weight in several ways. Cinnamon slows down the emptying of your stomach thus giving you an ongoing feeling of fullness. This helps prevent hunger pangs.

Cinnamon improves blood sugar metabolism which means your body will more readily break down sugars to serve as fuel for your energy needs. This means your body will have less unused blood sugar to store as body fat.

As cinnamon is a natural antibiotic, gut health will improve through adding cinnamon to your diet as it reduces the number of bad bacteria in the gut. A specific type of bacteria known as clostridium difficile has been found to be a contributory factor in causing obesity. The active component of cinnamon, which is called trans-cinnamaldehyde, can help get reduce these types of bad bacteria.

Cayenne Pepper

Cayenne is known for its compound named capsaicin. Capsaicin has the ability to fight obesity by helping the body reduce fat tissues and lower levels of blood fats. It also triggers protein changes in the body that results in reduced fat buildup.

Its thermogenic effect provides heat that allows the body to burn more fats as fuel. Research shows that a consumption of foods that have a thermogenic effect can help boost the body's metabolism up to 5%. It also improves the body's fat-burning ability up to 16%.

Capsaicin has been found helpful in counteracting the tendency for metabolism to slow down during the weight loss process. It assists in achieving steady and healthy weight loss over time.

Ginger

Ginger is beneficial for improving a person's digestive system as it regulates the movement of food from the stomach to the intestines. Ginger helps promote feelings of satiety which decreases the urge to binge. These actions are highly effective in helping a person to lose weight gradually and naturally.

Ginger is also a natural appetite suppressant which makes it an added boon for individuals wanting to lose weight.

Ginger contains vitamin C which is an antioxidant. As such it aids in detoxification, helps improve the body's ability to eliminate wastes and works to prevent fluid retention.

Add ginger to your shopping list as this is one herb for weight loss you don't want to be without. As well as adding ginger to your cooking you may even enjoy eating a piece of fresh ginger on its own.

Turmeric

Turmeric is used for many health issues, including unwanted weight gain and high cholesterol levels. These two problems are usually found in conjunction. Turmeric has lipid lowering properties which means it can be helpful for lowering bad cholesterol levels.

Similar to capsaicin, turmeric has a thermogenic effect which promotes fat burning. The curcumin content of turmeric also has anti-angiogenic properties that lead to a reduction of fat mass while inhibiting the growth of fat tissues.

Adding Beneficial Herbs to Your Diet

After reading about these different herbs, have you decided what you are having for dinner tonight?

Whatever you do, don't think that cinnamon laden donuts are an item you can add to the list. It's all about the foods you start with and the herbs added to those foods. Think healthy first and then add your desired herbs for improved weight loss.

Conclusion

Those with little awareness of herbal medicine are usually amazed at the range of issues that can be successfully treated by it, and that it is not only used for minor or trivial conditions.

It is worth remembering that many pharmaceutical "products" are only synthetic replicas of an herbal solution that has always worked. Maybe the synthetic version was developed due to natural availability limitations, or was it simply because the natural solution could not be patented?

If the herbal treatment works, why look elsewhere? You will be less likely to suffer unwanted side-effects, and less likely to have to take another pill to overcome the side-effects of the first one.

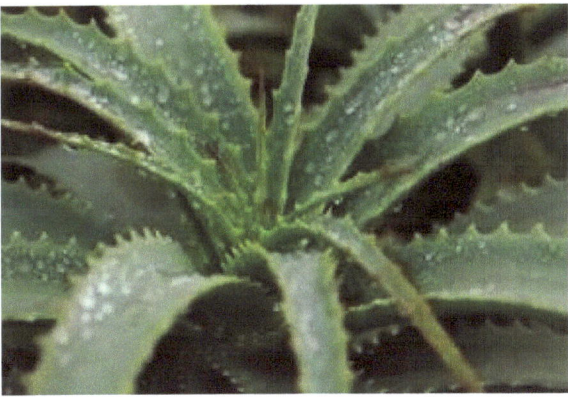

Glossary of Herbal Terms

There are a variety of herbal terms used by those familiar with herbal treatments, especially those involved in prescribing or dispensing. Some terms may have fairly obvious definitions, but others may seem quite obscure.

Here is a glossary of terms that will be helpful when researching and sourcing herbal preparations. Following most definitions are some herbs that are useful in performing that function. Please note there may be many other herbs that could be listed in each category, but only a few are listed for each.

Alterative: Blood purifiers that work to detoxify the blood and the lymph while promoting renewal of body tissue.

Blue Flag Root, Queen's Delight, Burdock, Ginseng, Chaparral, Marigold, Garlic, Echinacea, Devil's Claw, and Goldenseal.

Anti-Catarrhal: Herbs that reduce mucous production.

German Chamomile, Comfrey, Mullein, Witch Hazel, Garlic, Fenugreek.

Anti-Coagulant: Agents helpful for keeping the blood flowing easily and preventing platelets from clumping together or clotting.

Lime flowers, Ginseng, Garlic.

Anti-Emetic: Herbs that quell nausea and prevent vomiting.

Meadowsweet, Black Horehound, Chamomile, Nutmeg, Cinnamon, Dill and Cloves.

Anti-Infective: Remedies to stimulate the immune response in the body and help withstand infection.

Vitamin C, Echinacea, Goldenseal, Wild Thyme, Garlic, Red Clover, Holy Thistle.

Anti-Tussive: Agents used to relieve coughing, clear the lungs and lessen expectoration.

Pleurisy Root, Mullein, Angelica, Thyme, Slippery Elm Bark.

Antioxidant: Scavengers of free radicals within the body, compounds that protect the body from lipid peroxidation and from free radical activity.

Gotu Kola, Beet tops, Alfalfa, Garlic.

Anti-Lacteal: Herbs to decrease breast milk production, utilized for weaning a baby off the breast and drying up the mother's milk supply.

Sage, a common ingredient in turkey stuffing and the reason why nursing mothers' may have a hard time producing milk after Christmas and Thanksgiving supper.

Anti-Inflammatory: Agents that reduce inflammation by working to enable tissues to return to their normal functioning as opposed to suppressing inflammation.

Bio-Strath formula, nicknamed the "anti-inflammatory formula" contains a blend of the following herbs: *Echinacea, Horseradish, Marigold, Arnica, Balm, Hypericum, Bryony* and others. *Comfrey* is specific for bone inflammation, *Devil's Claw* for muscles; *Turmeric, Feverfew and Chamomile* are general anti-inflammatories.

Anti-Lithic: Herbs utilized for dissolution or elimination of gravel or stones. *Parsley Root, Gravel Root, Stone Root, Hydrangea and Pellitory of the Wall.*

Anti-Microbial: Plants with the capacity to inhibit the growth of micro-organisms and disease causing bacteria.

Mountain Grape, Buchu, Barberry, Camphor, Clove, Cinnamon.

Anti-Pruritic: Herbs that help to relieve intense itching.

Marigold, Chickweed, Cucumber, Peppermint, Chamomile.

Anti-Rheumatics: Herbs that can ease the pain of arthritis and rheumatism.

Celery seed, Wild Yam, Dandelion, Blue Cohosh, Lavender, Black Cohosh.

Anti-Spasmodic: Plant medicines that bring relief of mild pain, spasm or muscle cramp.

Lobelia, Dong Quai, Black Haw, German Chamomile, Valerian, Passion Flower.

Bitters: Bitters are a class of herbs that stimulate the bitter taste buds located in the back of the mouth. When this occurs, a hormone is secreted into the blood stream which increases production of juices within the pancreas and the stomach.

Bitters are typically given approximately half an hour before meals. They work to assist assimilation and increase the appetite while reducing fermentation in the intestines.

Popular bitters include: *Centaury, Wormwood, Feverfew, Chicory and Goldenseal.*

Catarrh: When the mucous membranes become inflamed, excess mucous can be discharged. Catarrh is often the result of allergy, toxemia, dust irritation, ear infection, sinus issue or inflamed tonsils. It is also commonly caused by a high intake of sugar, starches, and dairy and white flour products.

Contra-indicated: Herbs that should not be taken with a certain medical condition or while taking specific medications, as they cause an unwanted reaction. For example, some herbs are not suitable and therefore contraindicated during pregnancy or lactation. If in any doubt, check first with your doctor or pharmacist prior to starting a new herbal preparation.

Decoction: An herbal preparation made from the woody parts of a plant such as the barks and roots. These dense materials are brought to a boil and simmered in order to extract the active constituents. Typically, a decoction is made in the ration of 1oz. of the crushed or cut material simmered in 750 ml of water until the total volume is reduced by one quarter.

Afterwards, it is strained and cooled and taken in divided doses throughout the day. Using a covered vessel is recommended to prevent the volatile components escaping. Plastic free or non-aluminum saucepan containers such as ceramic, stainless steel or earthenware are ideally used.

Demulcent: A soothing herb that is rich in mucilage and bland in taste; offering protection to inflamed or irritated mucous surfaces. It is considered to be an Herbalist's alternative to glycerine. *Slippery Elm, Marshmallow Root, Plantain, Oatmeal, Liquorice Root, Mullein, and Meadowsweet*, among others. Typically, a demulcent is almost always given in conjunction with anti-lithic herbs for stones to protect the surrounding mucosa as the stone passes.

Emetic: Herbs that induce vomiting; used for expelling poison from the system. Emetic therapy is not as popular as it was in the 1800's; however, it may still be used for various conditions such as jaundice, bilious attacks, dropsy, swollen testicles and acidity. Bitters are often given afterwards to restore the tone to the stomach.

Febrifuge: Anti-pyretic, anti-fever agents to reduce high body temperature. *Elderflowers, Yarrow, Raspberry Leaves, Cayenne and Boneset.*

Galactagogue: Herbs utilized to increase milk production in nursing mothers.

Examples include: *Cumin, Nettles, Raspberry, Goat's Rue, Fennel, Holy Thistle, and Agnus Castus.*

Liquid Extract: Considered to be the most concentrated form of an herbal preparation. Liquid Extracts are stronger than a tincture and the majority of them contain alcohol. They can be made in a variety of ways including: under pressure, evaporation by heat and cold percolation. Commonly, Liquid Extracts are taken in water.

Poultice: Poultices are made by using dried or fresh herbs, wrapped in a piece of flannel, a linen handkerchief or muslin bag and soaked in hot water. Equal parts of vegetable oil or honey can be mixed together with the herbs until they form a paste. *Tincture of Myrrh* is often used if there is any fear of infection.

Common poultices include: *Bran* for neuritis or sciatica, *Comfrey* for fractures and ulcers, and *Hops* for muscle pains.

Tincture: A concentrated liquid extract made from the soluble constituents of plants, seeds, barks, or roots in order to preserve their vital medicinal essences.

Tinctures can be made on a base of glycerine and water preparation or an ethyl alcohol preparation and can last for years.

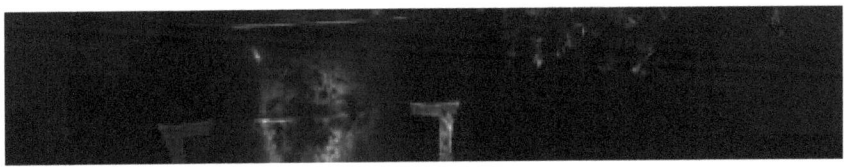

Other Relevant Books by This Author

If you would like to read more relevant books about this topic, here is a list of the CreateSpace links, titles and descriptions from this author:

https://www.createspace.com/5714434

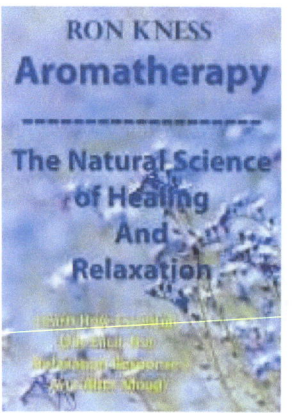

Aromatherapy - The Science of Healing and Relaxation

In my book, I reveal the natural holistic methods issues and to relive stress through relaxation.

In particular we talk about:
• Aromatherapy - what it is and how it works
• Essential Oils – how the effects of certain aromas differs from others
• Recipes – how to make your own essential oil combinations

Aromatherapy

The results of The American Psychological Association's 2010 Stress in America survey showed that nearly 75% of Americans who responded to the survey believe their stress levels to be so high that they feel unhealthy. Stress and anxiety reflect the reaction of the body and the mind when over stimulated.

Stress tends to reflect the physical responses of the body when coping with daily pressures, physical labor, a high-paced work environment, toxic relationships, and financial and emotional responsibilities, which exceed a person's ability to cope or manage.

However, your sense of smell can help relieve stress by smelling certain aromas.

Essential Oils

When selecting oils to combat anxiety and stress, choose oils with relaxing, calming, and uplifting properties. The oils should soothe while shifting the awareness in a way that grounds and replenishes the constitution of the person being treated. The scents that work best for anxiety and stress relief tend to have light and bright floral, citrus, or woodsy scents.

The essential oils recommended for relaxation and mood adjustment may be blended with those recommended for managing stress and anxiety. Many of them are complementary scents with complementary therapeutic qualities.

Recipes

There are many ways to enjoy the benefits of essential oils. When selecting a method of application, the issue being treated must be considered along with the desired results.

For example:
==> Creams, ointments, and gels work best for treating injuries like bruises and cuts.
==> A massage oil works well for treating muscle aches and pains.
==> If the primary purpose of the treatment is to shift a person's mood in some way, incense or a diffuser may be the best option.

While you can buy certain combinations of oils, we include in our book several recipes and show you how you can make a unique essential oil tailored just to you.

Aromatherapy – The Science of Healing and Relaxation is a must-have book for those that are overstressed and starting to exhibit the effects of stress either through the development of physical or mental responses, or both.

What you smell can make you feel better!

https://www.createspace.com/6414998

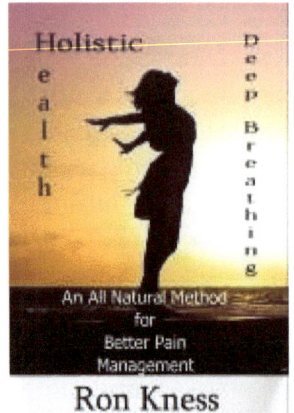

Deep Breathing to Help Relieve Chronic Pain: An All-Natural Method for Better Pain Management

Chronic pain is pain that lasts longer than six months and can't be cured, but can be treated and managed. The pain can range from mild to excruciating and can be either episodic or continuous.

According to WebMD, approximately 100 million Americans alone suffer from chronic pain; imagine the numbers worldwide!

Chronic pain can affect anyone at any age, for example, if you have a sports injury at a young age, the pain can sometimes follow you throughout life or you are 60 and diagnosed with arthritis … the stage I'm now at in my life having been diagnosed with osteoarthritis five years ago.

Often early injuries, present injuries, or other reasons end up causing chronic pain. Some people have certain genetic codes predispose them towards having chronic pain.

There are several conditions that cause chronic pain such as fibromyalgia, arthritis, neuropathy, carpal tunnel syndrome, migraines, and others.
You can also have an injury when you are younger and have chronic pain stemming from it but starting later on in life.

Chronic pain can be a result of repetition in body movement from a job and sometimes, people simply suffer from chronic pain syndrome whose cause cannot be identified.

Regardless, it can have a mind of its own, flaring up for no apparent reason with science still not fully understanding why.

So the best treatment is to try and manage it. While many try medications, sometimes their side effects are worse that the pain they are trying to manage. Others go for a more holistic method of treatment like deep breathing. It is cheaper, can be done anytime, doesn't have harmful side effects, and in some cases can be just as effective.

In this book we explore how deep breathing can reduce the effects of chronic pain along with the other health benefits of deep breathing.

https://www.createspace.com/6419369

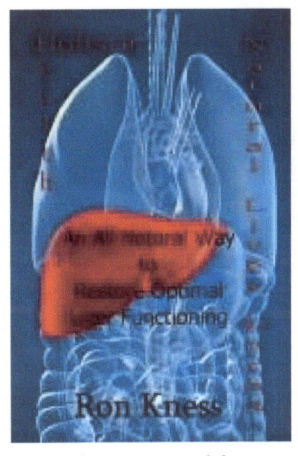

Natural Liver Detox: An All-Natural Way to Restore Optimal Liver Functioning

We live in a world that is chocked-full of toxins be it in the air we breathe, our food, our water… so much so that their entrance into our bodies has become unavoidable.

Exposure to these toxins requires that all of the organs in your body work in synergy to maintain homeostasis - meaning everything needs to be in a certain balance in order to function optimally. If the function of one organ or system goes awry, the others will also be affected.

Your liver and kidneys play a vital role of filtering toxins out of your body, but your liver has an additional function of breaking down the present toxins in order to expel them from your body.

This enzymatic process occurs in two phases – breaking down the toxins and bonding these broken parts to other molecules that destroy the toxic substances and expel them from your body through sweat, urine and fecal matter.

When the liver becomes overburdened or overworked due to chronic exposure to toxins via the environment, diet, smoking, alcohol use, lack of sleep or poor stress management, it can slow down and cause a back-up of toxins in your system. This can impact many other systems and organs in your body resulting in various symptoms.

In this book we show you the signs that your liver may be struggling, how to set up a detox plan and the foods to eat to help keep it operating at optimal efficiency.

https://www.createspace.com/6433160

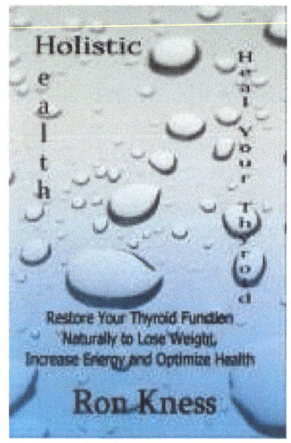

Heal Your Thyroid: Restore Your Thyroid Function Naturally to Lose Weight, Increase Energy and Optimize Health

The thyroid is a gland that is responsible for regulating many of your bodily functions and if it isn't functioning properly, you will experience a variety of symptoms that can impact your life in unfavorable ways.

The problem is that diagnosing a thyroid disorder can be difficult because the symptoms can be vague and attributed to many different things. Because of this, millions of people wake up every day with thyroid issues without even knowing it.

Do you constantly feel so fatigued that you barely have the energy to brush your teeth?

Do you find that there is more hair than usual ending up in your brush or shower drain?

Are you gaining weight or just not losing no matter how much you try to adapt a healthy lifestyle?

Do you often feel cold or have sensitivity to cold temperatures?

Do you have constant brain fog or memory issues?

Do you have dry eyes?

Well most of us experience these things at various times and because we simply assume that age is catching up with us or that we are not exercising as frequently as we should or that we are not getting enough sleep…we just chalk them up to something we have to live with and don't pursue any medical follow-up.

Many times it is an under-performing thyroid that is causing problems. With the proper nutrition, exercise and some lifestyle changes, you can heal your thyroid. They are all things you should be doing anyway, so what do you have to lose?

About the Author

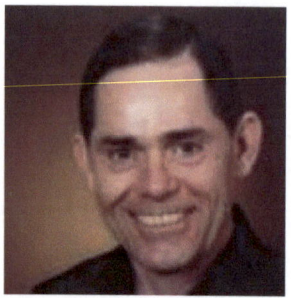

I have published over 125 books on Amazon for Kindle, CreateSpace and other publishing platforms.

While most of my books are on health and fitness in general, as I age (now 65) at the time of this writing) my topics of interest are geared toward aging baby boomers and older.

Besides my own writing, I also ghostwrite ebooks, books, reports, articles, blogs and do Kindle conversions for clients on a variety of topics.

Today my wife and I are retired from our careers and live in Gold Canyon, AZ. I now write as a retirement business where you'll find me happily sitting in my office typing away on my laptop as I work on my next book or ghostwriting project . . . that is if we are not traveling on a cruise ship - our new-found mode of travel.